STUDENT-FRIENDLY COOKBOOK

Cheap, quick, and healthy meals. Delicious, time-saving recipes on a budget

ELIZABETH FLOURNOY

DISCLAIMER NOTICE

TABLE OF CONTENTS

INTRODUCTION

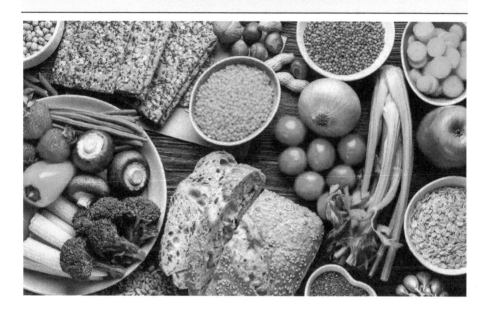

<u>Why Cook in College?</u>

Each FALL, HORDES OF understudies much the same as you leave the commonality of their folks' homes and main residences and show up on school grounds, prepared to move away from their secondary school days and progress into the grown-up world. For most, this implies living endlessly from home unexpectedly, meeting new individuals from better places, and starting to consider what sort of a vocation they may need. Not many, in any case, consider the way that their new residences don't come total with individual cooks. Presently your family's kitchen at home has been diminished to, best case scenario, a solitary hot pot that connects to the divider, or, best case scenario, a shared kitchenette that may just contain machines as complex as a two-burner oven and a toaster.

Regardless of what your experience, school will be a learning experience for you. You may wind up figuring out how to do logarithms, or figuring out how to do clothing. Yet, whatever you're considering, you'll need to eat, and that is the place where this book comes in. While you may think cooking has a place at the lower part of your school daily agenda, reconsider. Above all else, cooking is less expensive than eating out. In case you're presently liable for taking care of yourself (or part of your own particular manner), you realize that your cash is preferable spent on educational cost over costly eatery checks. What's more, don't believe you're free on the off chance that you live at home and go to a neighborhood school. You'll presumably find that your wild timetable doesn't line up with your family's eating times, and your folks will probably be not able or reluctant to go on kitchen obligation at 12 PM. Another preferred position to cooking is that it's more advantageous than eating out. Why is eating well so significant, you inquire? A decent eating regimen expands your capacity to deal with the anxieties of school life. Eating nutritious suppers at ordinary occasions encourages you rest better, gives you more endurance, and makes it simpler to oppose sugar-stacked bites that briefly raise your glucose levels yet leave you feeling more drained than any time in recent memory an hour later. Preparing more advantageous suppers at home will likewise assist you with evading the weight pick up numerous understudies insight in their first year of school: the feared rookie fifteen. At last, remember that cooking is entertaining! Spending Sunday evening in the kitchen is an extraordinary method to loosen up following a feverish seven day stretch of considering, and dominating new abilities gives you a feeling of achievement.

Remaining Healthy in College 101

Venturing out from home for school presents difficulties just as circumstances. In case you're somebody whose kitchen expertise doesn't stretch out past the warm setting on the microwave, learning essential cooking abilities alongside analytics can appear to be overpowering. It's all around very advantageous to surrender to the draw of the feasting lobby or food court. Nonetheless, the essential tips in this section will help change cooking from a task into an innovative, peaceful break from examining.

The Infamous Freshman Fifteen

Measurements show that roughly 50% of all understudies put on somewhere in the range of ten and fifteen pounds during their first year of school. Yowser, isn't that so? It's anything but difficult to succumb to the first year recruit fifteen when you're attempting to change in accordance with a bustling timetable and there's inexpensive food readily available wherever you look. Notwithstanding, gaining weight will simply build the pressure that you're now feeling from scholastic weights, and it very well may be difficult to take off later. Fortunately, there are approaches to fend the pounds off, and they do exclude restricting yourself to a bowl of plain oats for breakfast, lunch, and supper. Most importantly, adhere to a customary dinner plan. On the off chance that you are arranging a long report meeting ceaselessly from the dormitory, plan sound tidbits to take with you. Straightforward snacks, for example, Peanutty give energy without the fat and calories in potato chips and chocolate. Additionally, attempt to design your suppers about seven days ahead of time. One alternative is to cook ahead, making all your week by week suppers throughout the end of the week. It's a lot simpler to adhere to a sound feast plan on a bustling weeknight when you should simply warm up supper as opposed to setting it up without any preparation. At last, set aside effort to work out. Numerous universities have fantastic exercise offices directly nearby that are free for understudies. With a bit of arranging, you can fit an activity meeting into your day by day plan. An every day swim or oxygen consuming exercise makes it simpler to control your weight, and it additionally lifts your spirits by delivering endorphins, giving you a truly necessary increase in energy.

Flintstones Vitamins Don't Cut It Anymore

Clearly, dodging the green bean fifteen is a valid justification to eat well and deal with your body while you're in school, however it's not by any means the only explanation. Food isn't just about how your body looks outwardly; truth be told, it's the manner by which your body glimpses within that is generally significant. Thus, it's a smart thought to get to know the rudiments of nourishment to comprehend the fuel part of the food you eat. As such, things like nutrients, minerals, protein, calcium, and so on and so forth. Above all else, it's essential to attempt to try not to eat prepared nourishments at whatever point you can. School is maybe the most troublesome climate in which to do this, yet it is conceivable—and the advantages are many. Attempt to consistently pick the entire nourishments that are finished as nature proposed them. Prepared nourishments, for example, grains, sugars, and flours are regularly deprived of their common supplements. In any event, when nutrients and minerals are added back in later—a cycle called "advancing," which implies that the supplements lost during refining are added back in to improve the item—the complete impact is rarely the equivalent.

Setting Up Your College Kitchen

You can't cook even a container of soup without the correct hardware, so the initial phase in your journey to turn into an extraordinary school cook is to take stock of what you have as of now and make a rundown of what you need. Obviously, what you at last de-cide to carry with you to school will differ as indicated by your very own circum-positions. For instance, living arrangements with mutual kitchens regularly give pots, dish, and other cooking basics for inhabitants. Some school kitchens, then again, are just outfitted with the more fundamental apparatuses, for example, a toaster, wherein case there would be no reason for burning through cash on a rock solid skillet. In this way, considering your own kitchen circumstance, audit the accompanying arrangements of fundamental things and blend and match as per your necessities:

Bowls, Pots, And Pans

- A few blending bowls for consolidating fixings and serving noodle and plate of mixed greens dishes

- A few great pots and dish of different sizes

- A plastic or metal colander for depleting washed, whitened, and bubbled food

- One metal treat sheet for heating treats or heating up rolls

- One or two glass preparing dishes for use in the broiler

Utensils And Tools

- One or two wooden spoons for mixing a lot

- A heatproof elastic spatula for blending fixings and turning food during cooking

- A few great blades, including a serrated bread blade, a sharp hacking blade, what's more, a little paring blade

- A plastic or wooden cutting board for cutting, hacking, and mincing food

- A vegetable peeler

- A can opener

- A grater for grinding, destroying, and cutting cheddar and different nourishments

- A wire race for whisking eggs and sauces

- A set of estimating spoons

- A set of estimating cups

Some school living arrangements permit understudies to keep little electrical apparatuses in the dormitory or the home kitchen. A coffeemaker permits you to have some java prepared when you get up toward the beginning of the day. Tea consumers will need a pot for bubbling water. Alongside a toaster oven or toaster, these things will help cause your living quarters to appear to be more similar to home. With regards to bigger apparatuses, unquestionably consider a microwave if your financial plan and school guidelines license it. Despite the fact that it can't totally supplant a standard electric broiler, a microwave can be utilized for everything from making popcorn to setting up a whole supper. Minimal microwave and fridge blends, planned explicitly for quarters, are additionally benefit capable. Some even accompany a little cooler appended.

Eggs Benedict

This is a high-protein breakfast that will give you energy for the duration of the morning. This formula serves 4, so make certain to welcome a couple of companions over to go along with you.

Fixings | SERVES 4

- 3 tablespoons skim milk

- ½ cup low-fat mayonnaise

- 4 eggs

- 4 cuts bacon

- 4 cuts entire wheat bread or 2 entire wheat English biscuits

Staggering Edible Eggs

Eggs give a colossal measure of protein and next to no sugar, and they cause you to feel full. You ought to have one egg a day, yet recall that endless things we burn-through every day as of now contain eggs. Before you have your every day portion of egg, ensure your different suppers and bites don't contain an excessive amount of egg or you could try too hard.

1. Blend the skim milk in with the mayonnaise and warmth in the microwave for around 40 seconds to warm.

2. Break each egg into individual microwaveable dishes, being mindful so as not to break the yolks.

3. Cover each bowl with saran wrap and microwave on high until the whites are cooked and yolks firm, around 2 minutes.

4. In a skillet, cook the bacon.

5. Toast the entire wheat bread cuts and spot the bacon on top.

6. Add the eggs on the bacon and top each egg with 2 tablespoons of mayonnaise blend.

PER SERVING Calories: 295 | Fat: 20 g | Protein: 13 g | Sodium: 739 mg | Carbohydrates: 16 g | Fiber: 2.8 g

Egg White Bruschetta

This is an extraordinary breakfast to share at an early daytime gathering or to appreciate without anyone else. Add two additional cuts of bread to spread out the bruschetta on the off chance that you need to serve more individuals.

High-fiber, Vegetarian

Fixings | SERVES 2

Ingredients

- 7 egg whites

- 4 entire eggs

- 1 cleaved tomato

- ½ cup hacked mushrooms

- 1 little onion

- ¼ cup new basil

- ½ teaspoon salt

- ½ teaspoon pepper

- 4 cuts entire grain bread

Guidelines

1. Beat egg whites and eggs together.

2. Warmth hacked tomato, mushrooms, and onion in an enormous skillet. Add egg blend and scramble. Add basil, salt, and pepper as you scramble.

3. Toast bread and top with the egg combination.

PER SERVING Calories: 395 | Fat: 13 g | Protein: 34 g | Sodium: 1192 mg | Car-bohydrates: 39 g | Fiber: 6.6 g

Spinach and Ricotta Mini Quiches

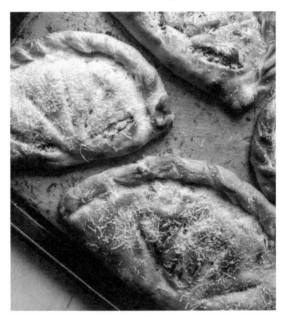

Top these small quiches with a cut of tomato and sprinkle on some destroyed cheddar to add a pleasant hint of shading and extraordinary flavor.

Low-calorie, sans gluten, Vegetarian, Low-carb

Fixings | SERVES 5

Ingredients

- 10 ounces cleaved frozen spinach

- 2 eggs

- 1 cup skim ricotta cheddar

- 1 cup low-fat destroyed mozzarella cheddar

Guidelines

1. Preheat broiler to 350°F. Spot cupcake liners in 12-opening cupcake tin.

2. Warmth spinach in microwave as indicated by bundle headings, until delicate and warm.

3. Whip the eggs and add the spinach. Mix together. Crease in the ricotta and destroyed mozzarella cheddar.

4. Fill each cup with egg-spinach combination, about ½" per cup. Heat 30 to 35 minutes.

PER SERVING Calories: 175 | Fat: 10 g | Protein: 16 g | Sodium: 273 mg | Carbohy-drates: 5 g | Fiber: 1.8 g

<u>Eggs Florentine</u>

You can supplant the mayonnaise with nonfat yogurt. This formula is especially acceptable with nonfat vanilla yogurt.

Veggie lover

Fixings | SERVES 2

Ingredients

- 2 English biscuits

- 2 eggs

- 5 ounces hacked frozen spinach

- 1 tablespoon low-fat mayonnaise

- 1 teaspoon salt

- 1 teaspoon pepper

- 2 teaspoons destroyed low-fat cheddar

Frozen spinach to the Rescue

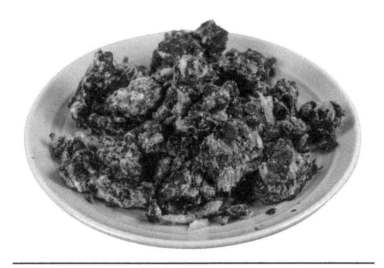

Frozen spinach is an incredible thing to have available. Simply purchase a few bundles all at once and haul them out at whatever point you're in a dilemma. It warms up rapidly in the microwave or in a griddle, and afterward you have a simple, nutritious element for omelets, sandwiches, side dishes, and that's only the tip of the iceberg. Look out for additional plans in this book that call for frozen spinach, for example, Spinach and Ricotta Mini

1. Preheat stove to 350°F. Spot biscuits on a preparing sheet.

2. Break an egg onto every biscuit. Prepare for 10 minutes.

3. In the interim, heat the spinach in the microwave until delicate and warm, around 2 minutes.

4. Add low-fat mayonnaise, salt, and pepper to spinach. Mix together.

5. Eliminate biscuits and top with the spinach blend. Add a teaspoon of destroyed cheddar and serve.

PER SERVING Calories: 260 | Fat: 10 g | Protein: 15 g | Sodium: 1621 mg | Car-bohydrates: 31 g | Fiber: 4.3 g

Chive and Cheddar Omelet

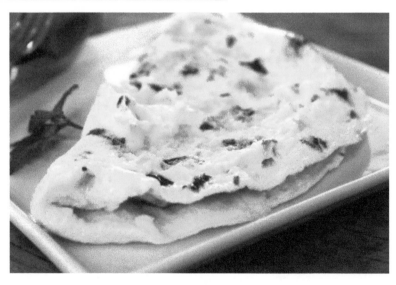

Chives are a great spice since they can be bought all year and will keep in the cooler for extensive stretches of time.

Veggie lover, Low-calorie, sans gluten, Low-carb

Fixings | SERVES 2

Ingredients

- 4 huge egg whites

- 1 huge entire egg

- ¼ teaspoon salt

- 1 tablespoon olive oil

- ¼ cup decreased fat destroyed cheddar

- 2 tablespoons cleaved new chives

<u>Magnificent Omelets</u>

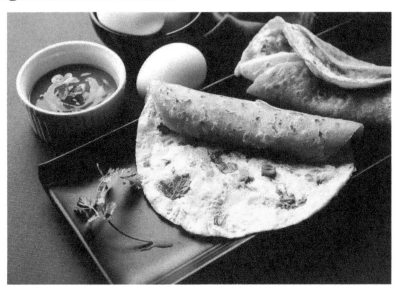

The phenomenal thing about omelets is that you can stuff them with a wide range of things. Different veggies, natural products, and cheeses make delectable mixes. Brie cheddar and cut turkey, or mushrooms and onions with Swiss cheddar, are two or three mixes you may pursue your next omelet.

1. Beat the egg whites and egg in a little bowl. Blend in the salt.

2. Warmth the olive oil in a little skillet on low warmth.

3. Pour the egg combination in to cover the surface.

4. Cook egg combination until edges show solidness.

5. Sprinkle the cheddar uniformly over the egg combination, and afterward do likewise with the chives. Overlap one side over the other.

6. Flip the half-moon omelet so the two sides are equitably cooked.

PER SERVING Calories: 156 | Fat: 11 g | Protein: 14 g | Sodium: 1392 mg | Carbohydrates: 1.5 g | Fiber: 0.075 g

Very Veggie Omelet

Change this formula by cleaving up any vegetable you like and adding it or subbing it for the peppers.

Low-calorie, without gluten, Vegetarian, sans lactose, Low-carb

Fixings | SERVES 2

Ingredients

- 4 huge egg whites

- 1 huge entire egg

- ¼ teaspoon salt

- ½ cup cleaved red peppers

- ½ cup cleaved green peppers

- ¼ cup cleaved onions

- ½ cup cleaved mushrooms

- 1 tablespoon olive oil

Guidelines

1. Beat the egg whites and egg in a little bowl. Blend in the salt.

2. Combine the vegetables in a little bowl.

3. Warmth the olive oil in a little skillet on low warmth.

4. Pour the egg combination in to cover the surface. Cook until edges show immovability.

5. Add the vegetable combination with the goal that it covers the whole egg blend equally. Overlay one side over the other.

6. Flip the half-moon omelet so the two sides are equitably

cooked.

PER SERVING Calories: 159 | Fat: 10 g | Protein: 12 g | Sodium: 442 mg |

Starches: 8 g | Fiber: 7 g

Wiener and Mushroom Omelet

In the event that you like a little zest, add a scramble of Tabasco sauce to kick up the flavor.

Low-carb, without lactose

Fixings | SERVES 2

- 4 huge egg whites

- 1 huge entire egg

- ¼ teaspoon salt

- 1 tablespoon olive oil

- ½ cup hacked cooked turkey frankfurter

- ½ cup hacked mushrooms

Turkey hotdog

Never knew about turkey hotdog? All things considered, it's time you did! Turkey frankfurter is an incredible, sound option in contrast to the standard assortment. Turkey is more slender and less oily than hamburger or pork, however it actually has all the incredible substantial goodness that you need in a warm breakfast or generous sandwich. Utilize cooked turkey hotdog in loads of assortments of omelets, sandwiches, dishes, stuffings, and then some!

- Beat the egg whites and egg in a little bowl. Blend in the salt.

- Warmth the olive oil in a little skillet on low warmth.

- Pour the egg combination in to cover the surface. Cook until edges show solidness.

- Add the wiener and mushrooms so they cover the whole blend equally. Crease one side over the other.

- Flip the half-moon omelet so the two sides are uniformly cooked.

PER SERVING Calories: 266 | Fat: 20 g | Protein: 20 g | Sodium: 631 mg | Carbohydrates: 2.5 g | Fiber: 0.34 g

Leafy foods Quesadillas

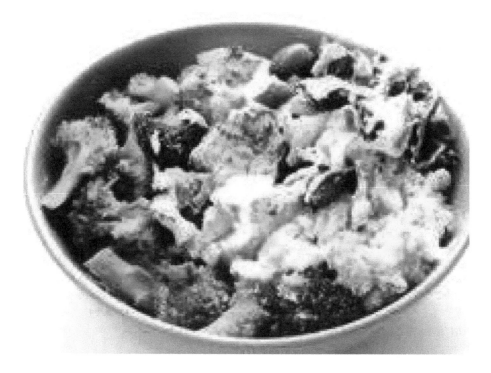

Insipid mozzarella is an ideal setting for natural product, and you can shift the leafy foods as per what's occasionally accessible. These are blade and-fork quesadillas, excessively gooey for finger food.

Veggie lover
Fixings | SERVES 4

- 4 tablespoons strawberry jam

- 4 (6" to 8") entire wheat flour tortillas

- 2 cups destroyed mozzarella cheddar

- 1 cup diced new strawberries in addition to extra for sprinkling

- 4 tablespoons strawberry yogurt for embellish Confectioners' sugar for cleaning

Magnificent Quesadillas

Much like omelets, quesadillas are one of those nourishments that can arrive in a wide assortment of flavors. This morning meal quesadilla incorporates leafy foods, and you can trade out the mozzarella cheddar and strawberry jam for whatever other sorts that you like. An extraordinary lunch quesadilla may have sautéed vegetables and hummus, and you can likewise make a supper quesadilla with Tex-Mex fillings, for example, barbecued chicken, dark beans, salsa, and cheddar.

At the point when quesadillas are on the menu, let your creative mind go out of control!

1. Spread 1 tablespoon jam on a tortilla and sprinkle it with ½ cup mozzarella cheddar and ¼ cup diced strawberries. Overlay over the tortilla to encase the filling. Rehash with the leftover tortillas, mozzarella, jam, and strawberries.

2. Splash the skillet with nonstick cooking shower and warmth it over medium warmth. Cook the quesadillas, each or two in turn, until brilliant on the base, around 3 minutes. Flip over and cook the second side until brilliant and the cheddar has liquefied.

3. Top every quesadilla with a touch of yogurt, a sprinkling of strawberries, and a cleaning of confectioners' sugar. Serve hot.

PER SERVING Calories: 380 | Fat: 16 g | Protein: 17 g | Sodium: 530 mg | Carbohydrates: 42 g | Fiber: 3 g

Prepared French Toast

This dish is incredible when presented with cut pears or peaches as an afterthought. To improve it further you can sprinkle a tablespoon of sans sugar maple syrup across the top.

Veggie lover

Fixings | SERVES 2

- 2 eggs

- ½ cup skim milk

- ½ teaspoon ground cinnamon

- ½ teaspoon vanilla concentrate

- 1 tablespoon powdered sugar

- 4 cuts bread

Guidelines

1. Preheat stove to 400°F.

2. Beat eggs and skim milk gently in a bowl. Add the cinnamon, vanilla, and sugar.

3. Absorb the bread the egg blend and spot on a nonstick preparing sheet.

4. Heat for around 10 minutes or until brilliant.

PER SERVING Calories: 253 | Fat: 8 g | Protein: 14 g | Sodium: 360 mg | Carbohy-drates: 34 g | Fiber: 2.8 g

Oats Buttermilk Pancakes

To make these hotcakes without sugar, substitute Splenda for the sugar.

Low-Calorie, Low-fat, Vegetarian
Fixings | SERVES 6

Ingredients

- 1 cup uncooked oats

- ½ cup flour

- ¼ cup sugar

- 1 teaspoon preparing powder

- 1 teaspoon preparing pop

- ⅛ teaspoon salt

- 2 cups low-fat buttermilk

- ¼ cup Egg Beaters Butter-seasoned splash

Guidelines

1. Consolidate oats, flour, sugar, preparing powder, heating pop, and salt in a bowl.

2. Whisk together buttermilk and Egg Beaters in a little bowl. Pour combination over dry fixings and mix together until just mixed.

3. Pour ¼ cup flapjack hitter on a hot iron arranged with spread seasoned splash. Cook until bubbles show up and edges are earthy colored. Flip and cook until done.

PER SERVING Calories: 158 | Fat: 2 g | Protein: 7 g | Sodium: 183 mg | Carbohy-drates: 29 g | Fiber: 1.1 g

<u>Stuffed French Toast</u>

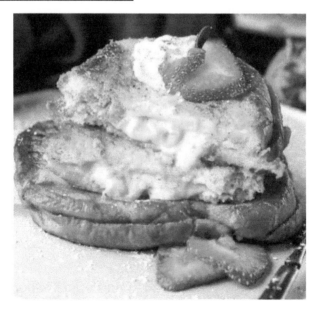

For this formula, make certain to cut thick cuts of bread. This will

make stuffing simpler, and you'll get extraordinary enormous cuts of stuffed French toast.

Veggie lover

Fixings | SERVES 4

Ingredients

- Spread seasoned cooking splash

- 4 1"- thick cuts French bread

- 4 teaspoons decreased fat cream cheddar

- 4 teaspoons most loved jelly

- 1 cup skim milk (separated into 4 servings)

- 1 teaspoon vanilla

- 1 teaspoon cinnamon or to taste

- ½ teaspoon nutmeg or to taste

<u>Trinity Variant-</u>

Hack up 1 green pepper, 1 tomato, and 1/2 a red onion. Put in a bowl and cover. This is your beginning blend that will go towards making 3 days worth of plans. a few things you can make with the blend:

Greek serving of mixed greens add some feta cheddar and some greek dressing, add some lettuce to give it more mass.

Spinach Salad-Put blend on a spinach serving of mixed greens, with a hard bubbled egg tossed in there for protein, and a few mushrooms.

Omelet-Add a portion of your blend to a couple of eggs. Blend it up, cook in a griddle, and add a touch of your #1 cheddar.

Prepared fish or chicken. Take some fish or chicken and put it in a preparing dish or container. Shower a touch of oil or margarine onto the meat, and add a small bunch of your blend ontop. Prepare in the stove.

Pasta: Add your blend to pureed tomatoes or alfredo sauce, and throw with your #1 pasta.

Rice-Cook a portion of your blend in the microwave for somewhat, at that point add some rice cooked in chicken stock.

Pan fried food Fry up your blend in with some meat or tofu. Add some soya sauce and put over rice.

Envelops Wrap up a portion of your blend by a pita or tortilla with some destroyed cheddar and discretionary meat.

Salsa-like item Add a decent scramble of new cilantro, some new parsley and white plant vinegar/lime juice, jalapenos and garlic, for something extremely stunning.

Bratwurst-Take a skillet, shower olive oil in the dish. High warmth. Toss some bratwurst in there and singe everything all sides until its earthy colored. Turn heat down to medium. Dump the green pepper, tomato and onion blend on to the skillet and afterward pour a dull lager in with it all. The measure of brew relies upon your skillet size. Go simply over mostly up your hotdogs. Cover the top and let those doggies steam for 30 minutes. Flip part of the way through. For the most recent few minutes you can eliminate the top and let the brew and veggie stock lessen to make a sauce. Serve on a toasted wiener bun with a little shop mustard and a portion of your decreased sauce.

Sautéed food:

Anything sautéed food is wonderful. Simply work on joining meats, veggies and flavors until you get a few suppers that you love. One of my favs is chicken, potatoes, spinach and onions with basil, garlic, pepper, red pepper, and salt.

In the event that you don't as of now, add streak singing to your sautéed food schedule. Just put oil in the wok, heat until it begins to smoke, throw garlic and ginger in, mix as quick as possible, at that point add the first of your fixings and continue like typical. The abrupt cooking adds a flavor to the oil that adds to the entire dish.

Another stunt is called going through. Actually I believe it's somewhat inefficient, I wouldn't suggest it except if you're cooking for a gathering. Fill your wok with enough oil to lower your meat completely. This is a decent an ideal opportunity to utilize a little wok and dainty cuts of meat. Warmth this until the oil begins to move around (indeed, this is somewhat frightening), dump your meat in, and mix. Eliminate the meat following a moment, strain it, and dump out all the oil you don't require for the remainder of the pan fried food. Add the meat back in later on. This seals the kind of the meat in, alongside the kind of any marination you utilized. It's awesome, yet that is a ton of squandered oil.

Cooked entire wheat fettucini blended in with a sautéed food produced using - cut onions, green beans, matchstick carrots, hacked ginger, teriyaki sauce.

Chicken and Rape-

you need to get: chicken, assault (it very well may be marked as "yau choy"), quail eggs, chicken eggs you likely as of now have: - a clean-ish pot - a dingy bowl you've eaten out of a couple of times - a grimy pan that you made eggs in or something - rice, sugar, soy sauce do these things:

1. start a pot of water bubbling. quit worrying about the minuscule bits of pasta adhered to it. those are beneficial for you.

2. throw rice and water in the rice cooker

3. put some soy sauce and sugar in the pan. they mix will with the spread from when you made eggs today.

4. water is bubbling, slash the chicken up and toss it in.

5. turn of warmth to pan

6. go mess around however long you like. rice producer close off consequently. you can't "over-heat up" the chicken.

7. come back, take the chicken out, toss it into the sauce skillet.

scoop a portion of the bubbling water into the foul bowl

8. while the bubbling water relax the tarnished bowl substance, kinda mix the chicken around in the container. wham, teriyaki chicken.

9. put chicken eggs in the as yet bubbling pot.

10. your bowl is currently perfect, similar to enchantment. Wipe it a piece, placed some rice in.

11. putquail eggs in the bubbling water.

12. move teriyaki chicken to capacity holder and put some on your rice for the impending supper.

13. throw the assault in the pot, placed the holder in the cooler.

14. cut the fire, placed the assault in the bowl with the chicken.

15. remove all eggs. result: you end up with: teriyaki chicken with rice and assault and a spotless bowl to eat them in, hard bubbled chicken egg for supper and some for some other time, hard bubbled quail eggs for nibbling, and a pot and skillet that confess all with simply a fast cleaning down. I have nourishment for quite a long time. entire cycle, beginning to end, took perhaps 20 minutes, with 10 minutes of game in the center. I additionally tossed like 20 messy forks, blades, chopsticks, and spoons alongside a scoop and spatula into the extra nearly bubbling water. they all confessed all in a split second when I washed them in the wake of eating. furthermore, the entire cycle just utilized one pot of water, so I am sparing the planet.

Chicken and Potato Casserole:

Get a bundle of frozen spinach, around twelve of those small infant red potatoes (the 1 or two inch ones), some dainty cut chicken bosom, and some montreal chicken flavoring.

Cut the potatoes down the middle—put the spinach at the lower part of a preparing dish. Put the potatoes in. Put the chicken on top. Sprinkle some flavoring on the top. Back at 350 for 45 minutes. Ensure YOU PUT FOIL OVER THE DISH!!

It takes around 10 minutes to plan and it is very delicious. Additionally, it is far superior for you than all the pasta/rice dishes recommended here. Living on pasta is an awful thought except if you are running A LOT or attempting to store extensive layers of fat for winter.

Dal:

There may be an underlying interest in flavors you might not have. Thereafter you're simply working through new vegetables, garlic, ginger and onions.

2 tablesoons ghee (on the off chance that you don't have explained margarine, you can presumably utilize olive oil) 1 onion, finely hacked 2 cloves garlic, finely slashed 1 inch piece ginger, finely chopped1 teaspoon salt 1 teaspoon turmeric powder .5 teaspoon paprika or stew powder 1 teaspoon coriander powder (get a modest mortar and pestle and granulate the coriander freshly)1 pound potatoes (washed and cleaved) 1 pound spinach 1 teaspoon garam masala (In Canada, you can get this at places like

Superstore, however as a single man it presumably isn't needed)

Warmth ghee and softly fry the onion, garlic and ginger Add the salt and flavors and fry for two minutes. Add potatoes and fry till half cooked. (The longest part) Meanwhile wash the spinach and hack finely.

Mix into the potatoes and keep broiling till delicate. Sprinkle with garam masala before worker Also: Lentils are bargain basement.

This is a delicious Dal, for vegans substitute vegetable stock, for the modest substitute water.

Quesadillas are a dietary staple.

Additional Sharp Cheddar, ground and two taco estimated tortillas (or one burrito measured collapsed fifty-fifty).

Spread one side of every tortilla, put one margarine side down in dish over medium/low warmth, layer with cheddar, crush in two or three bundles of taco chime gentle/hot sauce, cover with second tortilla adulate side. Cook until brilliant earthy colored, flip. Slice into triangles to make eating simpler.

Discretionary: layer within one tortilla with refried beans in a flimsy layer, place bean side down on cheddar and afterward margarine outside/top side so it browns when flipped.

96 hours of Chicken-

Night 1: Buy an entire chicken. Broil it, make sauce w/the skillet drippings and eat a thigh and leg w/pureed potatoes and a vegetable. Save bones.

Night 2: Take meat off chicken make a curry or sautéed food with a portion of the meat and a few veggies. Present with rice.

Night 3: Make tacos with left over meat

Night 4: Use the chicken stock that you ought to have made on day 2 to make a delightful chicken soup w/left over meat and other stuff.

Reward supper: take the wings off and split them so you have 4 pieces, heat up and throw in liquefied spread, garlic and hot sauce for yummy hot wings.

Enchilada dish

Fixings:

- Package of 10-12 tortillas

- Large jar of red enchilada sauce (hard to track down in Canada, simply in the event that you were pondering)

- 1/2 pound ground cheddar

- 1/2 onion

- 1 little jar of diced green Ortega chilies (whenever wanted)

- Large container of cut dark olives

- Vegetable oil

- 1 to 1.5lb of lean ground meat (or ground turkey; if utilizing ground turkey, season with loads of stew powder and dark pepper for additional flavor)

Bearings:

1. Dice onion, and sauteé in limited quantity of vegetable oil

2. Add ground meat, and cook until earthy colored

3. Drain olives, add to meat/onion combination

4. Add 1/2 would enchilada be able to sauce

5. Allow everything to stew on low for a couple of moments

6. Add wanted measure of diced chilies

7. Lightly fry tortillas in corn oil until delicate, and afterward channel on paper towels

8. Heat stove to 350 degrees

9. In ovenproof meal dish start layering meat blend, cheddar, and tortillas, utilizing 2-3 tortillas for each layer

10. Top with residual cheddar and enchilada sauce, and heat revealed for 20-30 minutes Best presented with taco sauce, acrid cream, and guacamole/avocados as an afterthought.

Chicken and Veggies

Boneless, skinless chicken bosom, some earthy colored rice and a green vegetable (broccoli, asparagus, Brussels sprouts, green beans, whatever).

You can grill the chicken or cook. Toss some salt and pepper on or get more extreme (teriyaki, garlic or lemon pepper, or bean stew sauce...) Boil or steam the veggies (I like mine firm).

Protip: Make a major clump of rice once every week and keep it in the ice chest to microwave when you need it. This can truly accelerate the time it takes to make this dinner.

You can generally trade out the chicken for a fish (I like salmon with nectar garlic dill sauce).

I have this for supper at any rate 3 times each week and think it is perhaps the most advantageous dinner around.

Meatloaf. Two pounds lean ground hamburger and a bundle of McCormick's Meatloaf Seasoning. You can purchase dispensable meatloaf dish or simply purchase an ordinary one. Portion skillet have LOTS of employments.

Follow the headings on the flavoring bundle. You will require eggs and milk. I don't utilize bread pieces or pureed tomatoes/glue. Individual inclination.

This cooks for one hour and you channel the meat at the brief imprint. Around then you can punch a couple of holes in the top and add a layer of pureed tomatoes so it will douse down into the meat or just spread a layer of tomato glue on the top.

At the point when you put the meat in the container you utilize your fingers to sort of form it into the corners and make the top level. Additionally, you can shape the meat on the base and sides leaving the center unfilled and fill it with cooked rice, pureed potatoes or cheddar for a 'stuffed' meatloaf and afterward utilize the remainder of the meat to cover the filling. Bode well? Extra meatloaf sandwiches are very delicious.

Hotdog Bacon Pasta Stuff

- Two or three segments of bacon, cooked and disintegrated

- 2 links of italian frankfurter, cooked and disintegrated

- 3 Tbsp margarine

- 1 garlic clove

- 2 Tbsp slashed parsley, Pinch each dried basil and oregano (I utilize Italian flavoring all things being equal)

- 6oz wine tool noodles

- 4 eggs, beaten

- 1/4 cup ground parmesan cheddar

- salt, pepper

Cook the meats, saved; soften the spread and saute the garlic. Add the bacon and hotdog, just as the flavors. Then, cook the pasta until done and channel. Add the pasta to the meat combination, mixing. Add the eggs and cheddar, mixing until the eggs coat everything and have started to set.

Helpless man's stroganoff

- Cook up certain onions and mushrooms in some margarine on the oven until delicate

- Brown up a pack of ground turkey or hamburger with garlic, salt, and pepper (Cayenne in the event that you like zesty)

- Add a container of cream of mushroom soup and a large portion of a cup milk

- Let stew, until it thickens

- Add sharp cream or eat with no guarantees.

- Put over rice or noodles

My idiot proof Chicken Enchilada/Tortilla Soup

Makes enough to take care of me for a few days so you can scale it on the off chance that you wish.

- 3 lbs-ish of chicken bosom or chicken or whatever

- 2 jars cream of chicken - modest stuff

- 2 jars unique Rotel

- 2 jars red enchilada sauce. (I utilize Old El Paso yet others may work)

- 2 jars dark beans (discretionary)

- Anything else you think sounds great. Perhaps hominy?

- Bag of mexican mix cheddar

- Cheap sack of tortilla chips

- 1 chicken bullion 3D shape

Cover the chicken with barely enough water to bubble it. Throw in the bullion block to enhance the stock a few.

Dice the chicken and eliminate some stock if there appears to be a great deal. You could keep it in a major bowl or cup and add it back in the event that you need more later. You don't need an excess of stock or it will weaken the kind of everything else.

Include all jars of stuff. Stew for some time to join everything.

Separate some tortilla contributes a bowl, add soup, add cheddar, Om nom

Modest, simple, solid sautéed food:

Slash up 1-2 cloves of garlic and toss in sautéed food container. Add 1-2 tablespoons of oil to get the garlic cooking (cook on medications high warmth for 1-2 minutes). Slash up one yellow onion to your ideal unevenness, add to the garlic and oil. Allow this to cook over medium warmth for a couple of moments until the onions begin looking somewhat straightforward. As you're cooking this, gradually add 1/4-1/2 cups of water to keep some dampness/juice in the base. Add a hacked red or green ringer pepper. Allow that to cook for one more moment or two. Add a cleaved zucchini. Cook for one more moment. Add a half square of tofu, cooked shrimp, chicken fingers or whatever other meat you might want/like. In any mix also. Anytime during cooking, don't hesitate to add pepper, salt, sriracha sauce, soy sauce, pan sear sauce, and so on

"Lancashire bacon and seared cheddar". (old however basic formula myfather showed me) Per individual 2 or 3 oz cheddar 2 strips bacon cut into matchsticks 1/2 16 ounces milk

Fry the bacon, channel the fat, decrease the warmth, add the milk, stand by a bit, add the cheddar, mix until the cheddar has softened, don't permit to bubble as it will coagulate. Present with dried up bread and dark pepper.

Simple sandwich chicken.

Required: 1 moderate cooker.

Fixings: 1.5-2 lb chicken 1 16 ounces ale Italian dressing dry blend

Dump it all in the moderate cooker. Meander back by after around 4 hours and shred. Cook about an hour after you shred it. Eat on rolls.

Pasta alla carbonara is extraordinary and modest. Simply heat up your pasta and cook it in a skillet with certain eggs, bacon, and pepper. Delicious, basic, fantastic.

Fish goulash.

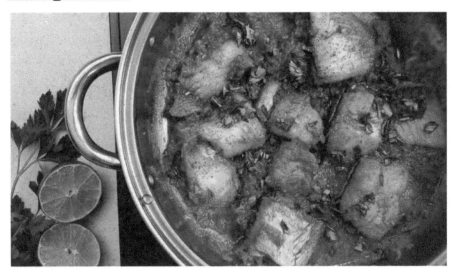

Little shell pasta, bubbled still somewhat firm (about a large portion of a pack)

- 1 can cream-of-mushroom soup

- 1 jar of fish

- whatever flavors you need to throw in modest bunch of destroyed cheddar

- modest bunch of white corn

I love fish goulash as well, however realized when I was truly in a bad spot monetarily that supplanting the container of mushroom soup with a white sauce (google the formula) and new mushrooms is path less expensive than the Campbell can. Haven't attempted the formula with white corn, however any corn would no uncertainty be less expensive local.

Since I'm in an ideal situation monetarily, I like to make the white sauce with white wine, garlic, and newly ground Parmesan or Gouda (or both) cheddar with lumps of new fish, shrimp, or turkey bosom ham. What's more, add a fragrant spice like new sweet basil, turmeric, or oregano.

Also, there are bunches of pastas that function admirably, some of which are somewhat costly. Possibly one of my next undertakings should be to figure out how to make custom made pasta.

Food Sludge-

Around 13 ounces of ground meat, a large portion of a pound of conventional high wheat oat (least expensive mass you can discover), one pound cabbage, one pound celery, one pound onions, one pound carrots, crush the vegetables, earthy colored the ground hamburger, put every last bit of it, including the oat, into a major pot and cover it with what seems like an excess of water and let it come down for around five hours, until you have a disturbing, unappetizing tanish muck. This should have the option to take care of you for around four days, one pound parcels for lunch and supper, half pound partitions for breakfast. The most ideal approach to gobble it is cook the bits. Like I stated, it's direction more muddled, however can be all the more fascinating and less expensive relying upon deals and where you search for the fixings.

Beans and Rice

were my staple in school (and now, that I have a new child)

Saute an onion, a lot of garlic, and a lot of peppers. I like pasilla (poblano) pepper, a red ringer, and a serrano. Start some rice, I like earthy colored rice-it's better for you, and I like the flavor and surface more. When the onion is earthy colored and delicate, put in a jar of dark beans. Put in the fluid, as well, it's yum. You can toss in a jar of tomatoes on the off chance that you like. You can likewise toss in some cumin, some cayenne pepper, some dark pepper, perhaps some salt. Possibly a hint of cinnamon, however truly just a squeeze. Make a poop ton and eat it throughout the week. You can likewise toss in a jar of corn. Avocado, wiener, acrid cream (or Mexican Crema on the off chance that you can discover it), sriracha, salsa, my significant other requests I state singed plantains, are largely your companions. Ooh, jack cheddar and cotija are acceptable. Also, cillantro. It's a pretty adaptable base, so you can switch things up enough to not become ill of it, and it's a finished protein and gets you the greater part of your minerals and stuff, eat some broccoli and corn and verdant greens to balance your minerals and nutrients.

Omelet.

Brisk. 2 or 3 eggs, one lubed frypan. Blend eggs in frypan in with fork.

Either top with nothing or with cleaved parsley, chervil, dried spices, ground parmesan cheddar, lotsa ground cheddar, BACON, cut mushrooms, truffles or straight conbination thereof. Eat from skillet, wipe frypan and set aside.

Dark Bean Loaf.

This is an exemplary vegan recipie that I love making, and typically turns out very well.

first step: cook some dark beans. Do this anyway you need. Actually, slow cooker short-term with garlic. Likewise turns out great to simply get a jar of pre-cooked bean. You need around 2 cups worth (1 can)

second step: empty the beans into a skillet with some oil, garlic, arbitrary flavors, whatever. I like mine fiery. Additionally very great with the "italian zest" shaker. Presently you will be crushing the beans while you cook them down. Plastic spoon or spatula functions admirably for crushing. Need to get it to the consistency of thick yogurt. This progression can take 10-20 minutes.

third step: blend the bean goo in with a cup(ish) of spaghetti sauce, two cups of breadcrumbs (flat bread that has been blendered), and two eggs. Add some more flavors here on the off chance that you feel like it. I ordinarily cleave up a clove or two of garlic and throw it in.

fourth step: prepare. 375 F for ~45 minutes, or until you don't want to stand by any longer. It doesn't generally should be cooked 100% of the route through, barely to cook the egg (160 F). Less time can be acceptable, yet additional time can likewise be acceptable. Changes the surface from more sauce-like to more meatloaf like.

The entirety of the estimations are from memory and I've utilized it with a wide reach.

Replacements can be made to accommodate your taste.

Reward round:

For the speedy, simple tidbit: Microwave omlette pita. Fill a half pita with daintily beaten eggs, cheddar, and hot sauce. Set it in a bowl so the pita doesn't spill. Microwave for ~1 minute.

Sunday morning frittata

4 potatoes-quartered... microwave 3 mins. the flip each piece and mic another 3 mins cut the potatoes into scaled down pieces add to non stick skillet with olive oil on medium hot warmth cook the potatoes season (salt and pepper) add hacked new broccoli , slashed red peppers, cuts of cooked wiener or ham.... throw and cook, add 6 or so beaten eggs... mix, flip... cook the combination... one eggs look nearly done mood killer the warmth add some ground cheddar (cheddar, mozzarella) a couple of sprinkles of tabasco sauce and you are in paradise

The world's best lentil soup

Fixings:

- 2 tsp cumin ground

- 1 onion (diced)

- 2 cups lentils (washed to eliminate starch and doused for the time being in water)

- 3 cloves new garlic (minced)

- 1 tsp basil

- 1 tsp oregano

- 1/4 - 1/2 tsp cayenne pepper

- 2 carrots (diced)

- 2 celery stems (diced)

- 6 cups of water

- 1 jar of squashed tomatoes/1/2 container of spaghetti (sauce tastes better some of the time)

- 4 bouillon shapes (enough for 8 cups stock, utilize chicken or veggie)

- 1 cup milk or cream (use cream)

- 1/2 cup of olive oil

TO DO:

- heat oil (on 8 or 9)

- add cumin and toast for 1-2 minutes

- add onion and garlic

- cook until onion is earthy colored

- add remaining flavors and celery, tomatoes and carrots, mix to cover

- cook for 5 minutes or somewhere in the vicinity

- add water, bouillon solid shapes and lentils

- cook 1/2 hour - 60 minutes, add milk/cream and serve

- Topping with lemon skin as well as cilantro

Fish Sauce Vegetables

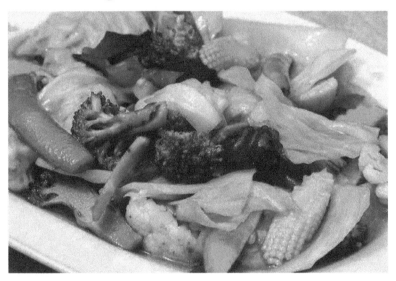

- Veggies from China town

- Fish Sauce

- brown rice

- fry them up

- Modest, can be made in like 10 minutes, and solid (toss some chicken in it each sometimes to celebrate)

Basic, modest, white truffle risotto.

Serves 4

2½ liters great chicken stock 50g margarine

1 onion, cleaved extremely, finely 400g superfino carnaroli rice 125ml dry white wine salt and newly ground dark pepper for the mantecatura: 75g virus margarine, cut into little dice about 100g parmesan, finely ground a white truffle 1 tsp truffle spread

A few hints: cleave the onions as finely as possible (the size of grains of ocean salt) - you don't need the onion to be clear in the completed risotto, and in the event that you have huge pieces, they won't cook through appropriately. Mesh the parmesan finely so it is immediately assimilated. Ensure that your spread is freezing. Cut it into little, even-sized dice before you begin cooking, and put it into the ice chest until you are prepared to utilize it. That way it won't soften excessively fast and it will emulsify as opposed to part the risotto. Keep in mind, the more rice you cook, the more noteworthy the warmth it will hold, so it will take less effort to cook.

To make the soffritto: put the stock into a skillet, carry it to the bubble and afterward decrease the warmth with the goal that it is scarcely stewing. Put a weighty put together dish with respect to the warmth close to the one containing the hot stock, and put in the margarine to soften. The decision of search for gold is significant, as a hefty base will disseminate heat equitably, forestalling consuming. As the margarine is dissolving, add the onion and cook gradually for around 5 minutes, so it mellow and gets clear, losing the impactful onion flavor, however doesn't brown - else it may add some consumed flavor to the risotto and ruin its appearance with earthy colored specks. I don't suggest that you add any salt now, in light of the fact that the stock that you will in a matter of seconds be adding will lessen down, concentrating its flavor. You will likewise be adding some pungent parmesan toward the end, so it is ideal to stand by until every one of these flavors have been retained and choose toward the end if you need any flavoring.

For the tostatura ("toasting" the rice), turn up the warmth to medium, add the rice and mix, utilizing a wooden spatula, until the grains are very much shrouded in spread and onions, and warmed through - again with no shading. It is imperative to get the grains up to a hot temperature prior to adding the wine. Add the wine and let it lessen and vanish, proceeding to mix until the wine has basically vanished and the combination is practically dry - that way you will lose any essence of wine. Starting here to the furthest limit of the cooking, for this amount of risotto it should take around 17-18 minutes (a moment or so less on the off chance that you are multiplying the amount). Begin to add the stock a ladleful at a time (each addition should be barely enough to cover however not suffocate the rice), mixing and scratching the base and sides of the skillet with your spatula. Let each ladleful of stock be nearly retained prior to adding the following one. The thought is to keep the consistency runny consistently, never allowing it to dry out, and to keep the rice moving so it cooks equally (the base of the skillet will clearly be the most blazing spot, and the grains that are there will cook more rapidly than the rest, except if you continue mixing them around). You will see the rice starting to grow and turn out to be more sparkly and clear as the external layer progressively delivers its starch, starting to tie the blend together and make it velvety. Keep the risotto percolating consistently at the same time as you proceed with the way toward adding stock, blending and allowing it to retain, at that point adding more stock.

After around 15 minutes of doing this, begin to test the rice. An expression of caution: let it cool before you taste or you will consume your mouth!

The rice is prepared when it is full and delicate, yet the focal point of the grain actually has a slight solidness to the nibble. At the point when you believe you are nearly there, lessen the measure of stock you are adding, with the goal that when the rice is prepared the consistency isn't excessively runny, however overall quite soggy, prepared to ingest the margarine and parmesan at the following stage and slacken up some more.

Take the dish off the warmth and let the risotto rest for a moment without mixing. For the mantecatura, immediately beat in the virus margarine, truffle spread, at that point beat in the parmesan. The outcome should be a risotto that is smooth, rich and emulsified. Now, taste for preparing and, on the off chance that you like, add a crush of salt and pepper, at that point shave over the white truffle. Serve the risotto as fast as could be expected under the circumstances, as it will continue cooking for a couple of moments even as you move it to your serving bowls (shallow ones are ideal), and you need to appreciate it while it is at its creamiest.

This should be a speedy prepare supper with a couple of replacements (as the quarters will frequently restrict your storeroom) on the fly. On the off chance that you can't accepting truffle spread in the feasting lobbies, simply purchase the fixings independently and make a compound margarine yourself. Maybe a completing spread would likewise get the job done?

Expectation I helped, great eats to you!

salmon prepared rice.

I just made one for supper, it's straightforward, modest and delightful.

Ingredients

- rice

- salmon filet

- cheddar for sauce:

- margarine

- a container of mushroom soup

- mushrooms

- onion

- broccoli and cauliflower

- a scramble of paprika, salt, pepper, any spices would be

pleasant as well, for preparing

1. cook rice

2. prepare sauce in an alternate pot, stick onion and margarine first. at that point everything else, mixing infrequently, let it stew for some time, and afterward season to taste

3. put rice in a broiler safe bowl, and afterward pour sauce on top of the rice

4. slice salmon filet and organize pieces on top of sauce

5. grate cheddar above, covering everything

6. stick bowl in a pre-warmed broiler, hang tight for 15 minutes, until all the cheddar has liquefied

Most effortless salsa ever (and tastes absolutely marvelous):

A huge container of diced/squashed tomatoes (16oz or thereabouts) a more modest jar of diced tomatoes with peppers (8 oz) 1/8 red (purple) onion (tighten up, cause an excessive amount of will ruin it) one bundle of cilantro Lawry's garlic salt (to taste - most likely around a Tbsp) Lemon juice.

2 Tbsp splenda (or sugar, however I'm attempting to keep it more beneficial)

Mix everything up in a food processor each thing in turn not to a glue, but rather to better particles. Blend in a bowl. In the event that you have all the fixings and a fundamental food processor, the entire thing can be made in under 5 minutes, is great, and will make you more appealing to a mate, and you will score higher on tests.

Bean Salad.

Hit up the canned bean segment of your supermarket and choose 3-5 jars of beans or corn that you might want in your plate of mixed greens. Dark beans, pinto beans, kidney beans, entire portion corn, green beans, chick peas, all work. Blend all these up into an enormous bowl, and some salt, pepper, or some cumin. This will give you alot of bean plate of mixed greens so whatever you don't eat, cover and put in the refrigerator, endures a decent week. At the point when prepared to serve you can eat it plan or add your number one plate of mixed greens dressing, hot sauce or whatever, be inventive.

Pan-fried food-

To begin with, begin heating up some rice.

At that point put some olive oil in a wok on high fire and put this in it:

- Assorted chicken pieces (wings, filet, anything goes)

- cook until salmonella-safe.

- Assorted vegetables (normally accessible stowed and precut).

- A LITTLE soy sauce.

Turn down the warmth, and mix a decent measure of Boursin through it all.

Add the rice, make the most of your feast

Facon. Next time you make some bacon spare the oil in your ice chest. Get some tofu, and fry it shortly of the oil. The kind of the tofu is so impartial it gets devastated by the greatness of the bacon. On the off chance that you utilize a large portion of a shape of tofu for the formula, this expenses around 50 pennies to make.

Couscous

.This can be made in huge clumps - couscous - knorr chicken stock blend (the powder kind) - I generally eyeball the stock to couscous. take a gander at the water needed for both to get a smart thought

Blend these in a tuperware holder. Add any or the entirety of the accompanying: - pistachios - cumin - apricots (cut up) - bean stew drops - raisins - red lentils - thyme - whatever

Presently you should simply take out the sum that you need and add water. This is useful for a speedy lunch to go and is super chirp. Couscous is preferred for you over ramen noodles. In the case of making at home, sprinkle with olive oil.

Pruned Chicken

Ingredients

- 4 chicken filets, diced

- 1 pack (250 grams) of dull dried prunes slice to bits

- 1 tin (250 grams) of dark olives, cut

- half a container (50 grams) capres (depleted)

- fresh green pepper grains to taste

- 100 ml olive oil

- 100 ml dark balsamico vinegar

Let this marinate a few hours (or shockingly better: overnight) in the cooler.

Put in a broiler dish and cover freely with aluminum foil. Cook in the broiler for around 30 minutes at 180 degrees celcius.

Meanwhile cook some pasta, light the candles and pour the wine. A solid, dim red wine presumably suits best.

Thai Curry

Thai red curry glue and thai green curry glue are the two best things you can place in your ice chest. The subsequent best is chicken sauce (Sriracha hot pepper/bean stew sauce in a plastic jug with a chicken on it). Simply ensure you purchase the huge containers of curry glue in chinatown, not the stuff you can discover in little westernized containers in the supermarket which costs an excessive lot of cash.

Fast and scrumptious curry:

Heat up oil. Add hacked onion, some curry glue, and bean stew peppers on the off chance that you need (dried ones turn out great). Toss in a jar of coconut milk (under $1), a drop or two of fish sauce (in the event that you need, discretionary), some lime juice (have a major compartment of the bundled stuff in your cooler on the off chance that you would prefer not to need to purchase limes each time you make this, however limes are likely less expensive/better), and water. Work it up, add more glue on the off chance that you need to, possibly some oil on the off chance that you need that, and afterward toss in hacked vegetables (bok choi, carrots, celery, bamboo shoots, peas, whatever) and cook until they're finished. You can make the sauce watery with loads of coconut milk, water, and lime, and it resembles a watery thai curry, or you can make it more like a thick sauce so you have to a greater degree a sautéed food sort of thing. Serve on rice.

Another other option, and less expensive:

Make rice. As the rice water is bubbling, toss in some curry glue, nutty spread, lime juice, slashed onion, fish sauce (simply a sprinkle), and some earthy colored sugar on the off chance that you need. To this you can add vegetables, hacked pork (you can use around 1/3 to 1/2 pork cleave, to get a touch of meat in your eating regimen without going through a great deal of cash), or cooked fish (for a little while I utilized frozen salmon which I had found on special, which I just microwaved - who cares if it's intense, it's going into tacky rice curry and it mellow and gets flavourful there), shrimp, whatever you feel like or have found at a decent cost. Cook until the rice is delicate and the meat is finished.

A modest, yet unspicy thing: Cook rice. In the last stages, toss on top a lot of slashed peppers, onions, broccoli, and pork or whatever other meat you've found at a bargain and put in the cooler. Put the cover on and the food gets steamed on top of the rice.

Heavenly and simple.

At long last, and this one is pretty accursed acceptable: cherry grill chicken. 1 can pitted dark cherries, a cup of grill sauce, cleaved chicken. A touch of hot sauce is a smart thought here, in the event that you like zest. Toss every one of the three fixings (counting the juice from the cherry can) into a pot and cook until done on medium or thereabouts. Serve on bread or egg noodles. You can make a similar dish with pork.

Make nice estimated groups of any of these things and for a couple of bucks you'll have in any event three or four dinners worth.

Hand crafted Falafel

2 cups dried chickpeas 1 medium onion, minced 5 garlic cloves, crushed 1 cup new cilantro, hacked (you can utilize parsley in case you're not a cilantro fan) 1 tsp preparing powder 2 tsp newly ground coriander 2 tsp ground cumin ½ tsp red pepper drops 1 tbsp genuine salt ½ tsp dark pepper Vegetable oil for browning

Cover the chickpeas with water and splash for 24 hours. Channel and put in a safe spot.

Utilizing a food processor, beat the chickpeas until they finely cleaved yet not child food. You need it to look like breadcrumbs. Add the onion, garlic, cilantro, preparing powder, coriander, cumin, red pepper chips, salt and pepper to the combination. Cycle until the fixings are joined and the combination is a light green. It should at present be a grainy surface.

Note: If you have a little food processor, this may must be done in clusters.

Eliminate the blend and cautiously turn out 1" balls. These will feel like they will self-destruct, however they won't... I guarantee! Try not to exhaust them, this isn't care for making meatballs. Delicately structure them and spot them on a sheet dish.

While the falafel is chilling, heat an electric fryer or an enormous pan with oil. The oil should be about an inch down and around 350 degrees.

Tenderly drop the falafel into the hot oil and fry for around 3-5 minutes - they will be overall quite brilliant earthy colored. Eliminate and spot on a paper towel lined plate to deplete. Serve falafel on pita bread with lettuce, tomato, red onion, cucumber and your ideal sauce(s).

Heated Chicken Parmesan

4 boneless skinless chicken bosoms or identical chicken strips 1/4

cup softened margarine

1/2 tsp garlic powder (or most likely two or three minced garlic cloves) 1 Tbs Dijon mustard 1 tsp Worcestershire sauce 1/3 cup bread morsels 1/3 cup ground Parmesan cheddar 1/8 cup dried parsley

Combine the margarine, garlic powder, Dijon, and Worcestershire in a dish. (I normally utilize old pie searches for gold.)

Blend the bread pieces, Parmesan, and parsley together in another.

Dunk the chicken in the spread, at that point in the bread scraps, at that point place in a buttered or lubed 9x9 or so dish. Prepare at 350 for 50-an hour, until done through.

Heated Chicken with root veggies.

Get a Whole Chicken...Un-wrap it and burrow inside to take the Giblets out-

They ordinarily come enveloped by paper and stuffed inside the crude winged creature. Flush the fowl with Water and afterward pat dry...as dry as could be expected under the circumstances. Utilize your finger to isolate the skin from the breast...don't remove it however separate it to make a pocket...and then stuff incredible things in the pocket. I typically toss in whatever new spices I can get at the market and some garlic. Completely margarine or oil the outside of the offer and salt and pepper it. Do a harsh slash of all your veggies...anything just slice to generally a similar size - Potato, Baby Carrots, Onion, Parsnip. Put the Veggies in the preparing dish put the chicken on top with the bosom side up and put the dish in the over at 500 for 20-30 mins. Turn the over down to 425 and keep heating for 60 minutes. The planning time for this should take around 15 mins and when it is done you will resemble a brilliant lord of cooking. By staying the wiped off and afterward oiled up fowl in the burning hot over, you singe the external keeping all the dampness inside.

On the off chance that YOU DO NOTHING ELSE...DO THIS

Purchase a little pepper and salt processor. They are not modest, but rather that $6 speculation will most recent a year. You can purchase renditions of all your #1 spices with the processor incorporated into the top, in practically any market nowadays. Blended berry pepper newly ground makes eating an egg an occasion - The red, green and dark pepper join into a gathering in my mouth. DO IT.

Greek Salad

Fixings:

Ingredients

- 2 medium measured tomatoes

- Half red onion

- Half green pepper

- 50-100 grams feta cheddar, more on the off chance that you like it:D

- Half cucumber

- Olives

- Olive oil

- A little Oregano (like half teaspoon)

Cycle:

1. Cut the tomatoes in 4 pieces each, put them on the plate

1. Cut the cucumbers in rolls and afterward each move in two pieces

2. Cut the peppers and onions in stripes, rings are acknowledged, put them on top of the plate

3. Put the feta as an afterthought, or cut it in more modest pieces and put on top of the plate

4. Top up with certain olives

5. Add some salt in the event that you need (on the off chance that you do, its essential to add it before stage 6) 6. Add a little oregano Serve with bread.

Whatever else is definitely not A GREEK SALAD. Varieties exist and they are a subject of taste yet this is the first. For a more understudy benevolent variety, I don't utilize cucumbers, I don't utilize olives and in some cases not even onion. For my taste the fundamental fixings are tomato, feta and olive oil.

You can likewise add a container of fish on top of the serving of mixed greens to make a snappy and overall quite sound full feast. Try not to utilize oregano in the event that you add fish.

Make the most of your servings of mixed greens

Egg Fried Rice and Veggies:

$3 - Cook up some white rice, I generally start with 1cup of dry rice. When the rice is done saved it, don't stress in the event that it gets cold. Presently cook 2cups of frozen veggies, I ordinarily utilize the sort that arrives in a major pack (corn, peas, and carrots). When the veggies are done, channel them and put them in a safe spot. Presently put a teaspoon of vegetable oil in a skillet and warmth it drug high for 4mins. Add 3 eggs to the skillet and mix them around until they become pleasantly fried eggs. Presently put all the rice you cooked into the skillet with the eggs, mix it around until they are combined pleasantly. Presently add one teaspoon of minced garlic, and furthermore include all the veggies. Mix it all around for around 3 minutes. Done. This makes around 4 suppers, and by and by is extraordinary as an extra.

Macintosh and cheddar pizza-

What you'll require: Box of unique art macintosh and cheddar (should have the option to get it for something like 89 pennies for each container); Totinoz cheddar pizza (Publix sells them 3 for $5 and, for me at any rate, 1 pizza serves one effectively and turns out consummately for supper); destroyed cheddar (which actually type you like).

Fundamentally you bubble up some water and make the macaroni as taught on the crate, while making the pizza in the stove, or microwave, as educated on the container. When both have are cooked, you take a decent measure of the macaroni and put it on top of the pizza; enough to cover the highest point of the pizza without pouring out over the edges. You at that point take the destroyed cheddar and sprinkle it on top of the macaroni. This part is significant as the cheddar will liquefy and hold the macaroni together; you may likewise need to put a layer of cheddar howl the macaroni yet this isn't essential so I will leave this to your watchfulness. Presently for the undertaking of softening the cheddar on top; while the warmth from the pizza and macaroni might sufficiently be to do this without anyone else, what I did was stick the whole pizza back in the stove. Despite the fact that the stove ought to have been killed subsequent to taking out the pizza, the leftover warmth should be all that could possibly be needed to liquefy the cheddar and hold the macaroni set up. Leave it in there until the cheddar has liquefied equally so, all things considered it should be prepared to eat with no requirement for cooling. In the event that you utilized a microwave, simply make certain to warm it for something like 30 seconds so the cheddar has the opportunity to dissolve. you'll presumably end up with an enough macaroni left over to make another pizza should you like it, and you can undoubtedly refrigerate it and use it again at some other point.

Blend pound in with broccoli-

Fixings

- 2 Potatoes

- 3 Carrots

- A tad of ground cheddar, and a little milk (for the pound). Something like gentle cheddar, your least expensive cheddar, it's simply adding flavor.

- 1 Broccoli sprout

- Salt

- Olive oil (well you can do without however it's more advantageous, and adds excellent flavor).

- FRESH parsley, chives. You can abandon this as well, however it rocks to have it. :-) * Any kind of sauce that works out in a good way for pound. I like mushroom thick sauce, however you can likewise accomplish something basic like a half bubbled egg. If not, the feast might be excessively dry, yet unwind in light of the fact that it's still acceptable.

Alright so arrangement, simpler than dropping a huge load (uh oh, trust I didn't destroy your supper there... hehe).

Planning Okay, so I'll begin with a rundown of everything first: Boil potatoes and carrots. Crush the potatoes and carrots. Serve on plate with the broccoli and a fixing sauce.

Presently the long form: Peal the potatoes and carrots and wash them. Cut them in small pieces, extraordinarily the carrots, since you need them to bubble quick. You will squash them, so it doesn't make a difference how little, indeed, the more slender cuts of carrots the better. You can bubble carrots and potatoes together. Bubble them until they're soft, if the pieces are little it shouldn't take over 15 minutes.

While you're heating up the potatoes, separate the broccoli sprout into little cells and put into bubbling water. Broccoli needs to bubble just for around 5 minutes, since it shouldn't be exaggerated, it should be a piece crunchy, as are veggies. When the broccoli is done, channel it a little pungent spread to give it flavor, or simply salt. Another alternative is salt + olive oil. At any rate you get the essence.

Alright at this point the potatoes and carrots are soft, so channel them, add some margarine, 1 teaspoon olive oil, and a little ground cheddar, and start with a fork to squash the smidgens together. On the off chance that you bubbled them enough, it should be truly straightforward. The potato is the pound, the carrots won't crush just as the potatoes yet that is truly ordinary, it's simply offering surface to the squash (consider it crush with hacked carrots inside). You should hack the parsley and chives finely and add them there. OK, while squashing, you can change to a spoon once you see that it's as of now pound, and keep blending, until it's smooth.

Serve the pound with your preferred broccoli and the sauce. You'll cherish it. Exceptionally the squash.

PD: You can explore different avenues regarding the crush. Make it beautiful. Potatoes, hacked carrots, ground cheddar, garlic, and so forth At times you can take a touch of the bubbled broccoli and add it to the squash (you may have to bubble more) so it's yellow-orange-green... Scrumptious and substantially more intriguing than plain squash.

Medditeranean Salad

Essentially, a great deal of tomatoes, possibly three. Cut them into your ideal measured pieces. Gracious, and they should be delicious tomatoes, and cruncy. ñum ñummy... Did I say a great deal? OK much more since that is essentially it.

Presently a few olives, dark, earthy colored, green... add a small bunch of those.

Presently dress this plate of mixed greens along these lines (and in this specific request): Salt first, olive oil second, vinegar last (in the event that you like, not generally important). The explanation is that the salt goes very well with the tomatoes, however on the off chance that you put the oil first, at that point the salt won't get to the tomatoes as they'll be protected. In any event this is the genuine Spanish way.

In the event that you like, you can slash garlic and parsley to add flavor, however not all that much.

My Ever Evolving Vegetarian Chili Risotto

Start with a jar of Diced Tomatoes

- Add any blend of Bean, Lentil, Chickpea

- Add any kind of Rice

- Any Spices you may like

- Add more vegetables. Beets, potatoes, carrots, onions, spinach, lettuce (essentially anything)

- Add some meat like thing. I've been utilizing tofu as of late. You could likewise utilize meat, however ensure you sort out some way to cook it just prior to blending it in.

- Add whatever other fascinating nourishments you may need in it: Raisins, Nuts, Balsamic Vinegar, More Spices, Boullions Cubes.

You cook and mix until everything appears to be cooked, about 20 minutes. I'm by and large adding fixings the entire time that I am causing it, to aside from possibly the most recent 5 minutes. Serve it with ground cheddar on top, or curds directly close to it. You can put it on toast in the event that you like.

I have likewise given putting ground chocolate a shot it, which was very delightful.

The way in to this formula isn't to follow a formula, simply go with your gut. I for the most part have enough for 4 or 5 dinners in the wake of making one cluster.

My overly mystery flapjacks formula:

- 1 cup self raising flour

- 1 cup milk

- 1 egg

- A spot of cinamon (in case you're feeling gutsy)

Stage 1: filter the milk and cinamon into a bowl

Stage 2: add the milk and egg, speed until all fixings are adequately consolidated

Step 3: on the off chance that you need slender hotcakes, blend in a touch more milk until the blend is more slender. In the event that you need thick flapjacks add a smidgen more flour and blend.

Stage 4: stand by a couple of moments until the combination rises.

Stage 5: pour some combination onto a buttered frypan at a medium warmth. Make it whatever size you need. On the off chance that you need excessively flimsy flapjacks, move the frypan around with the end goal that the combination while still uncooked spreads out across the frypan.

Stage 6: flip the flapjack with a spatula once bubbles begin showing up. cook until you can see the underside is cooked.

Stage 7: top with your number one garnishes, lemon squeeze and sugar, or jam and cream are acceptable.

Stage 8: rehash with the remainder of the blend. The blend will likewise save well in the refrigerator for a day, so you can utilize it the following morning, however will require some all the more blending.

Lentil Stuff-

One of my top choices for fast, simple and modest: 1 c dried earthy colored lentils (washed and picked over for rocks and terrible beans), 1.5 c hacked tomatoes and juices (canned is fine), 1 c water or stock, 1 onion, slashed, 2 tsp minced garlic, 2 T olive oil, 1 tsp each ground cinnamon, tumeric, and cumin, 1 cove leaf

Warmth oil in a pot, add onion and cook for 5 minutes, blending. Add garlic and flavors and cook for one more moment. Add lentils, tomatoes, narrows leaf, and water or stock, halfway cover and cook, mixing incidentally, until lentils are delicate (25-30 minutes), adding extra fluid if important to forestall consuming (should be sassy instead of soupy).

You can twofold this formula and make lunch for an entire week for around 5 dollars! Extras freeze truly well, as well.

Eggplant Strips-

- 1 or 2 Eggplant (This is your "meat") - cut the long path into strips.

- 1 white onion. (Dice)

- 1 red onion (Cut off the finishes and cut into 'rings', at that point cut down the center so they are "C" molded.)

- 1 or 2 loads of cilantro. (Dice)

66

- 4 to 6 Roma tomatoes. (Dice)

- Lawry's Garlic Salt (blend in as cooking, not all that much) and

- Lawry's Seasoning Salt (Or Johnson's, on the off chance that you need to kick in an additional dollar or two) Get a sensibly measured skillet and pour in some vegetable oil. Add these fixings and mix.

You can likewise add different veggies that suit your extravagant (Bell peppers, Jalepenoes) yet this is the least expensive and most straightforward form.

In the event that you need to twofold the costs, you can drop the eggplant and get a pound and a portion of chicken or skirt steak. Cut into long strips and add to the skillet defrosted. Perhaps let the meat cook for around 5 minutes before you put veggies in.

Expectation you like it. It took care of me many spending plan tight evenings, and gave me some cool focuses with the vegan young ladies who were intrigued that I could make veggies taste so nummy.

Creamless cream of whatever soup:

- 1 onion, slashed

- 2ish potatoes, slashed

- about the potato's volume in some sort of vegetable, slashed, broccoli is acceptable.

- bouillion blocks or goo

In a major pot, sautee the onion in oil until clear. Add the potato, vegetables, water to cover, and a few bouillion blocks or spoonfuls. Stew until the potato is cooked.

Whenever bouillon is disintegrated, taste for in the event that it needs more flavah, add more bouillion assuming this is the case.

Permit to cool, at that point mix to perfection.

Improvements for taste: hacked garlic, different spices n' flavors, some additional cream or yogurt prior to serving. Spread or bacon oil rather than oil, shallots rather than onion. Enhancements for cost-adequacy: frozen vegetables are commonly less expensive than new. Or then again for new, watch out for what's on special. This soup freezes extraordinary, so keep some tupperware around and spare a bundle for when you don't have time or tendency to cook. Start glancing in the cooler when you are eager.

Prepared Chicken-

Simply get a few breadcrumbs, olive oil, and some chicken bosoms (and, maybe, anything extra you may like - bean stew poweder, parmesan cheddar ... it's up to you.). Furthermore a delectable veggie - ie Asparagus or green beans (sugar snap peas are adequate, yet not as delicious - they lean toward searing for a more limited timeframe).

Discover a dish with adequately high sides. Wash the chicken bosoms, and afterward rub down with some olive oil. Spoon a portion of the breadcrumbs onto the two sides of chicken, at that point place on (oiled) skillet. Coat veggies in olive oil, and afterward sprinkle salt and pepper to taste - mastermind around the chicken. In skillet, cook this for roughly 45 minutes at 200 (345 F) degrees celsius.

After this, eat your delectable, scrumptious veggies and chicken. Truly, this crap is delicious as damnation.

Swabian Potato Salad (my top choice) 4 huge, bubbled potatoes, When cooled, strip and cut them dainty (If conceivable favor waxy potatoes for making a plate of mixed greens. Coarse potatoes may break while cooking.) 200 ml hot meat stock (or vegetable stock) 1 tsp mustard 1 little onion, finely cleaved 1 tbsp wine vinegar 1 tsp sunflower oil salt, white pepper as per your taste

Combine: vinegar, oil, mustard, onion, salt and pepper 1 tbsp. of meat base with 1 cup high temp water. Pour the fluid combination over the potatoes and blend altogether. Make the most of your serving of mixed greens! The potato plate of mixed greens tastes best when it is still somewhat warm.

Celebrated pork hacks

Earthy colored pork hacks and onions in skillet with olive oil. Add 1 jar of cream of celery soup + 1/4-1/2 jar of water. Cook on low until pork is delicate and soup looks less like cream of celery soup and more like sauce. Present with moment pureed potatoes or white rice. City Chicken Season cubed pork with salt and pepper, dig in flour and earthy colored in skillet with olive oil. Move to broiler verification dish, add 1 jar of french onion soup and heat at

475 for 35 minutes, at that point sear for 10. Then again you could simply add the french onion soup to the skillet and diminish heat until done.

Potato Hobo Pack-

Purchase frozen, diced potatoes with cleaved peppers previously remembered for the pack. Pour a portion of the potatoes onto a bit of tin foil. Add a large portion of a stick of margarine, wanted flavors, and (this is significant) about a large portion of a cup of brew on top. Close up the tin foil so it is a selfcontained liner. Set broiler to sear, cooking time fluctuates with load, yet generally around 25 minutes. They taste screwing remarkable, and since potatoes are exceptionally high on the satiety file, they top you off. Likewise, you can get a pack of diced potatoes for like $2, and one sack will make in any event three suppers. Expansion of vegetables and other stuff is discretionary - I like to imagine that is the thing that the brew is for, however that is simply me.

Microwaved egg sandwich-

I want to eat this with entire wheat bread, yet any bread will do. Typically, for an egg sandwich, you would sear it, yet it is a lot simpler (and more advantageous) to pop an egg into an artistic bowl, pop the bowl in the microwave, and cook for one moment. The egg comes out steaming and cushioned, and is anything but difficult to eliminate from the bowl with an utensil. Drop the egg onto your mayonnaised-to-taste bread, and appreciate.

Wiener and Bean Stuff-

- 1 clove garlic

- 1/2 cup hacked onion

- 1 lb smoked hotdog

- 2 cans spread beans (goliath lima will don't DRAINED lager discretionary: celery, ringer pepper, smoked paprika, dark pepper, ground chipotle some cooked rice

Cut the smoked wiener meagerly, and put into a skillet on drug low warmth. Slash the onion, add it to the skillet. Here, in the event that you need you may add two or three tablespoons worth of thinsliced celery and chime pepper, however they aren't important, so I didn't show them in the fixings.

Toss a cover on it, and let it go for 5 or so minutes, at that point mix. Rehash. Presently add the garlic. You should cut it flimsy, at that point slice it the alternate method to make bits. It works better to it this route in this dish than to utilize a press.

Give it a mix, returned the cover on for five minutes.

At the point when the wiener looks overall quite dull outwardly and everything is delicate and done, wrench the warmth up to high. Allow it to warm up for a moment, however don't allow it to consume.

Pour in the lager, around 2/3 of a 12 oz brew is acceptable. Scratch, scratch, scratch all the dry stuff from the lower part of the container, and mix it as it cooks down. At the point when it comes practically down to nothing, add the spread beans(undrained. Try not to allow it to arrive at where things are beginning to stick.

When the beans begins to bubble, turn down the warmth to medications low. Cover, stew, mixing regularly. In around 5 minutes, the spread beans will start to separate and thicken the sauce.

Slop it over the rice. You will be astounded.

Tips and exhortation:

Utilize a brand of margarine beans that isn't "prepared". Karmas or Bush's Best(hate the name) are acceptable in my general vicinity. Check the fixings: no requirement for anything other than spread beans, water and salt.

Nature of the hotdog unquestionably has emotional effect on the nature of the dish. Notice that no salt was recorded, you needn't bother with any. However, it is some of the time ideal to add dark pepper, or smoked paprika, or both. I now and again utilize a little ground chipotle.

On the off chance that the frankfurter is extremely lean, utilize a tablespoon or two of bacon oil or olive oil. I entirely utilize a tablespoon of each.

You can begin the rice before you do whatever else. It will normally be done a little before the hotdog and beans, which is fine. Truly, 15-25 minutes ahead of schedule is fine, inasmuch as you keep a cover on it.

This isn't my ordinary way of cooking. I hauled it out of my butt once when I was in the temperament for Southern. I'm certain I'm not the primary person who could possibly do something like this. I was very amazed how great it was, and I ultimately enlightened my girl regarding it. It turned into a close family top choice at her home. At that point she disclosed to certain individuals... Long story short: every individual who attempts this formula joins it into their short rundown of ordinary things. It is simple, modest, fulfilling, nutritious and YUMMY.

For a genuine redneck party, do it with some stewed new collards and serve the entire thing with cornbread and sweet tea.

Potato soup.

Solid shape up 2 - 4 potatoes (depending how much left overs you need) to what in particular actually size you need, and afterward to do likewise for any veggies you need, I like to utilize onion and carrots generally. Add to a pot that has around 1 cup of milk and 1 table spoon of margarine per potato, or whatever appears to be acceptable, add salt, pepper, basil, sage (simply whatever flavors/spices sound great) and put onto medium - medium high warmth for around 30 - 45min (you'll need to check how delicate the veggies are around 30min, and afterward cook varying.) –

Scalloped potatoes.

Simply cut up 2 - 4 potatoes (the more slender the better, typically, they'll be cooked through simpler and in a more limited measure of time) and add whatever veggies you feel like, cut in any capacity. I like entire asparagus, cut onion, coarsely destroyed carrot, and so forth A few people like to set out a layer of tatoes in a heating dish, and afterward a layer of veggies, at that point potatoes, however I just typically blend them up and toss them in the dish. You'll need to cut up perhaps 6 stack of margarine, contingent upon how profound your dish is, and afterward space these similarly on top of everything. On the off chance that you have it, I urge you to put cheddar on top. Prepare on 350 for 45min - 1hr, or until cheddar is pretty cooked. My better half and I like these dishes in any case =]

Pasta Sauce-

1 container of tomato. Some new parsley. A smidgen of onion. A quarter carrot. A little bit of celery on the off chance that you have it. Salt and margarine. Fry the diced onion for 1-2 minutes in spread.

Add canned tomato (italian in the event that you can discover it, with nothing added - so no garlic, basil, and so on) + salt

Put in bit of carrot and celery (and a clove of garlic in the event that you wish, entire - this is only there for flavor and you take every last bit of it out prior to serving) Cook for 30-45 minutes, add parsley 5-10 minutes before done.

Present with pasta. Incredible approach to intrigue companions and expected lady friends, since it's actually that acceptable, and basically no work.

Satay sheep/Beef/Chicken with Rice

- Rice - 1 container of Campbells chicken soup - 1 bundle of Onion

Soup - Milk - Onions - Meat (Steak, schnitzel, is ideal, in any case Lamb, Chicken) - Peanut Butter - Seeded mustard (discretionary) First put rice onto cook

In another dish, - Cut meat and onions, fry in a container until cooked - Pour in jar of soup - Put onion soup bundle into can and load up with milk, blend - Add in 1 tablespoon of nutty spread and Mustard on the off chance that you are utilizing it - Pour Soup/Milk blend into skillet, mix - Cook for an additional 1 moment

Mood killer the meat/satay dish and trust that rice will cook.

Serves in any event 4, contingent upon the measure of rice/Cous

To utilize extra rice:

Pan fried food some meat (ham or chicken) until nearly done, add minced garlic and ground ginger for around 30 seconds, add the cold, clumpy rice from the ice chest, at that point when it's warmed through, throw in several whisked eggs and throw until the eggs are set.

Simmering pot Roast

Put a little modest dish or half meal cut into little pieces in moderate cooker. Add a cleaved onion, a cut carrots, a small bunch of pearl grain, hacked celery, cut tomato, salt and pepper (coarse pepper in the event that you have it).

For meat, add a half lager or a large portion of some water, a straight leaf and some thyme. For pork, add slashed new or some powder ginger and a cut apple or two, a large portion of some water.

Mix at that point cook on low for 6 to 8 hours.

In the event that you don't have or like pearl grain, placed diced potatoes in a few hours prior to eating.

Simmering pot chicken with cream cheddar

Put two bone-in chicken bosoms into a simmering pot with salt, pepper and an entire, entire pack of oregano, so much oregano you truly can't determine what's underneath. Add around 1/2" of water and turn the vessel on low and leave for 6-8 hours.

At the point when you return home from school, start a pot of rice. Eliminate then chicken from the pot and with two forks shred the chicken off the bone, at that point return it to the vessel with about a square of cream cheddar and a container of cream of something soup (mushroom, celery, whatever) and turn the vessel to high. Mix until it's overall quite rich, serve over the rice with a decent chianti and some fava beans.

Chinese Chicken Drumsticks:

Ingredients

- 1.5kg Chicken wings

- 1/4 Cup soy sauce

- 4 Cloves of Garlic

- 2-3 Tablespoon of Ginger ground (=about a solitary snapped off bulb)

- 1 Teaspoon every one of salt, pepper and sugar

- 2 Tablespoons mirin/rice wine/Sherry, on the off chance that you don't have anything great, cognac/rum works okay

- 2 Tablespoons canola/sunflower oil

- 1 Tablespoon Honey

Guidelines

1. Cut every chicken wing into three pieces, the wing tip, and the upper/front arm (Save wing tips for the soup as stock)

2. Optional: This is truly work serious however justified, despite any trouble, For the front arms with two bones, cut around the more modest bone and haul it out. For both the front arm and upper arm, snatch the more modest finish of the bone and cut around it however just 3/4 of the path down the bone. After this turn the meat back to front to shape a 'drumstick' with the wing. Photos of another formula, yet same technique for how to turn back to front

3. Mix all fixings above aside from chicken, for the marinade.

4. Put chicken wings in marinade for the time being (or 8+ hours)

5. Bake at a moderate temp (200'C), or on the off chance that

you just have the oven, add some water and put the blend on a low warmth in a pot with a cover. Both for ~40 mins

Ginger chicken soup:

Ingredients

- 4 Tablespoons of Oil

- 4-6 Tablespoon of Ginger ground (=about 2 snapped off bulbs)

- 1 White + 1 Red Onion

- 5 Cloves of Garlic

- 4 Celery Stalks

- About a modest bunch of finely slashed corriander leaves

- 1 Tablespoon every one of Salt, Black Pepper, White Pepper

- 6 Cups of Veggie Stock

- 6 Cups of Chicken Stock

- Wing Tips from previously

- 1 Kilo of chicken wings cut into 3 pieces

Guidelines

1. Crush garlic and finely slash alongside corriander

2. Chop onions and celery as you wish

3. In an enormous pan, toss oil in and fry garlic and onions for 3 mins

4. Chuck in everything else and cook for 40 mins on a medium warmth (shouldnt be bubbling) in an enormous pot

5. You now have a weeks worth of food, I trust you like chicken wings

Potato Soup:

Purchase a major sack of yukon gold potatoes, a pack of onions, olive oil, new garlic (in the event that you don't accepting new, try not to), cayenne pepper, salt, pepper, milk, flour, and chicken stock. Cook your potatoes well in the microwave and take off or keep the skin and shape or crunch contingent upon how much your like stout soup, cook your julienne (sp?) and minced onions and garlic in the skillet, adding the flavors after the warmth is off, at that point dump in your potatoes and onion poop in a major pot with your milk, chicken stock and around a few tablespoons of flour to make it thick. Measures of everything ought to differ as per the amount you like it. Estimations are for individuals that don't have the foggiest idea what they like.

Astonishing Burgers:

Purchase ground meat, an onion, a couple of new, red mellow peppers, cayenne pepper, pepper, salt, new garlic, frozen spinach, and either allegro steak sauce or a comparative kind relying upon your preferences. Cook and channel spinach, slash all your crap to your inclination, at that point add everything in to the meat as you would prefer. Keep in mind, an excessive amount of allegro methods your burgers will be excessively pungent. Flame broil flawlessly, at that point eat. These things can be cheap. From the outset when you're purchasing your flavor assortment, it WILL be expensive ($3/zest however salt and pepper are modest), yet consider them ventures. They'll last numerous suppers and you can tune things as you would prefer. Likewise, the fundamentals are noodles, canned beans, canned tomatoes, potatoes, flour, onions,n frozen spinach, and meat. A large portion of them are under $2 each aside from meat so while they have numerous fixings, they are genuinely modest.

Rice and Beans.

Make yourself a major pot of rice and beans toward the end of the week. Utilize the dried sort of beans and simply cook them in with the rice to make it somewhat simpler. You can toss somewhat salt in to make the water bubble quicker and give it somewhat more flavor. And afterward over time you can add anything to it.... veggies, chicken, tofu... Furthermore, flavors! (bean stew powder, cayenne pepper... anything goes)

Chicken Piccata.

Cook chicken, onion, garlic, mushroom, escapades, lemon, and tomato in a dish with some oil, salt, and pepper. I utilize 1 lemon for each 1 or 2 individuals served as a rule. A large portion of the lemon goes in while its cooking, half towards the end.

At the point when your normal chicken dish gets exhausting, this generally fulfills my quest for more flavor. Present with a side dish, broccoli, rice, or pasta.

Rice is likewise an extraordinary modest approach to eat. White rice is anything but difficult to make and keeps going forever. Simply take a few (ideally subsequent to being refrigerated for at any rate a night) and toss it in a dish to broil. Add anything you'd like, garlic, onion, pees, corn, broccoli, cleaved mushroom, even some cheddar on the off chance that you like, and scramble up an egg to toss in while its cooking.

Dark bean burger -

They are truly simple to make and are amazingly heavenly. It makes around 8 patties and expenses around $12 to assemble. I like muenster cheddar, ketchup, and pineapple on mine.

They cook truly well on a Foreman Grill.

1 can dark beans 1 can pinto beans (both depleted) 1 egg ~2t cumin ~2t stew powder ~1/4 t ground white pepper Half of a container of Kikkoman Thai stew glue 1-2 t sri-racha hot bean stew glue Chopped cilantro 1/4 cup Bread scraps

Pound beans with clench hand until around 2/3 of them are crushed up. Blend in any remaining fixings, adding bread pieces last. You may require somewhat more or less bread pieces. The blend should be firm. Refrigerate for a few hours prior to utilizing.

I recorded those brands for reference since they're regular to discover, I don't mean for an unobtrusive promotion. What's significant is that the Thai bean stew glue be the sort that has heaps of sugar, and the other is red peppers in vinegar for heat.

Straightforward goulash-

Get some elbow noodles, some sauce, and a pound (clearly this part acclimates as you would prefer) of ground meat. Cook each independently and toss it in a bigass pot. Put in whatever flavors you like, I will in general prefer to put a little stew powder and montreal steak preparing on the meat for some additional kick. A $10 pot of goulash will last you seven days. At any rate it's about $10 where I am for the fixings. Best part is that goulash is extremely, filling so even a little bowl will hit the spot. Something about carbs and meat just removes any appetite.

SHEPHERD'S PIE!!!

There are numerous plans accessible, however even this extremely straightforward one is scrumptious:

1.5lb ground hamburger (I utilized 93/7, 90/10 is acceptable yet don't get 80/20 imo) 1.5 bundles of moment sauce (the powder kind where you blend in water to make it yourself) 1 pack of blended veggies (I utilized peas/corn) 1 box of moment pureed potatoes (100% characteristic, taste great, endures like 3 of these pies)

Drop the hamburger in a skillet, you needn't bother with any margarine or oil, the fat melts and the meat cooks in it (this is the reason you don't get 80/20, it turns into a soaked wreck). When the meat is THOROUGHLY cooked (hamburger conveys heaps of germs and poo, take as much time as necessary and cook for some time over low warmth regardless of whether you believe it's done, cooking over low warmth won't dry it out like high warmth).

While you're trusting that that will complete, defrost the peas/corn. I just put them in a bowl with warm water, and put them through a colander when they weren't frozen any longer.

Additionally, make the pureed potatoes.

Get a dish. I utilized something like a 13" by 8" and it made very great pie. Spread the meat along the base. Pour in sauce, spread it. My better half and I added a tad of asiago cheddar, costly however screwing great. At that point put a layer of your peas/corn. At that point spread your pureed potatoes over the top, and possibly sprinkle some cheddar over them. Put it in a 400 degree broiler for like thirty minutes.

- It's tasty

- It keeps going numerous suppers... the above makes in any event six strong servings for about $15, and a portion of these fixings (like the crate of pureed potatoes) are reusable.

Yet, the BEST part is: - You CANNOT screw this up. Truly. You have different veggies? Toss them in. Chicken rather than hamburger? Concoct it, toss it in. Chicken sauce with ground turkey? Don't worry about it. Got an alternate sort of cheddar? Put it in. You can make this stuff in any request, it doesn't make a difference. The formula is EXTREMELY adaptable with adding various things, adjusting it, cooking things for various measure of time, you truly CANNOT screw this up. I scorn cooking and can't cook good for anything, yet I made tasty shepherd's pies. They're unfathomable.

Try not to eat them such a large number of suppers in succession or shepherd's pie loses its sorcery.

Hot Asian Peanut Butter Sauce for pasta. Modest, nutritious, simple, quick and extravagant enough to intrigue a chick with the expansion of a little side serving of mixed greens and white wine or Asian lager.

1. Use your blender to thin 2/3 cup of nutty spread (stout or not, your decision) with 3/4 water until it's the consistency of a slim sauce. You need it adequately thick to stick, yet thin enough to pour effectively - change pb or water varying, remembering that it will thin a small piece when it hits the hot pasta, at that point thicken altogether when it gets cold.

2. To this, add 3 Tbsp soy sauce, 2 Tbsp white or rice wine vinegar, 1 Tbsp nectar, 1/2 tsp ginger, and your capsaicin conveyance vehicle of decision to taste (ground stew powder, chicken sauce, new peppers, and so on) until it's zesty enough to feel it, yet not very hot. You simply need a decent kick in the rear of the throat and some glow in the mouth, not a "perspire and swear" Asian dish. Additionally the warmth will develop as it sits, so the extras are in every case fairly more sultry.

3. Blend until smooth and everything is fused. Allow it to merge while you cook the pasta. Twistings, raddiatore or some other shape with sauce-snatching little hiding spots are ideal, however you can utilize whatever you have.

4. If you have any frozen peas, broccoli or some other veg you love, throw it in with pasta when it's about done, sufficiently long to cook through. This adds some surface, shading and sustenance, however isn't essential.

5. Put depleted pasta (and veg) into a major bowl, pour sauce over the top and blend well.

Latkes

- 1 egg

- 1 tbsp flour

- 2 or 3 potatos (ground finely, as with a cheddar grater)

- 1/2 onion, slashed well

Combine it all, at that point fry in oil or margarine. I use around 2-3 spoonfuls of hitter for each potato hotcake. Eat em with ketchup, chutney, jam, whatever. Make sure to grind those potatoes well or they won't cook directly through!

Chicken with red peppers-

Dead straightforward and incredibly great. You need chicken, red peppers and soy sauce (I additionally hacked up a mushroom and tossed it in) preset broiler to 350 degrees. Put chicken in glass preparing dish, cut up red pepper (or whatever shading pepper is your inclination) and put it in the dish on top of and next to the chicken bosom. At that point pour loads of soy sauce all over everything. At that point stick it in the stove for 30 minutes. Incredibly great served over rice.

(Additionally great tidbit - take a rice cake and put cuts of cheddar on top and microwave it for 20 seconds. Eat warm. Astounding!)

pizza meal:

- 1 8oz box of elbow macaroni

- 2 cups destroyed mozzarella cheddar

- 8oz curds

- 1 12oz container pizza sauce

- 1/2 - 3/4 bundle pepperoni cut into equal parts. 1/2 tsp of basil

- Cook pasta dependent on bearings on box. Channel. Blend pasta in with the remainder of the fixings in 2 quart goulash dish. Sprinkle parmesan cheddar on top whenever wanted.

- Cover and Bake at 350 degrees for thirty minutes.

Microwave Directions

Get ready as above, however cover with cling wrap and stick it in the microwave for 7-9 1/2 minutes, pivoting midway. Ive never attempted to microwave it

Note: One you can sub or add to a wide range of things instead of the pepperoni. adding italian hotdog (earthy colored it first) has been pretty mainstream.

<u>Amazing and simple taco soup:</u>

- 1lb of ground turkey (I utilize 1.25 in light of the fact that that is the amount it's sold in)

- 1 enormous yellow onion

- 1 would kernel be able to corn

- 1 can pinto beans

- 1 can dark beans

- 1 can diced tomato with green stews

- 1 can Santa Clause fe beans

- 1 parcel of taco flavors. cut the onions up into little pieces, and cook them with a touch of oil. Add the turkey and cook that as well. At that point throw everything in a pot and warmth it up till it's warm. Makes around 6 truly filling dinners. You can put cheddar on it as well in the event that you need.

I for the most part make it on Sunday, and freeze what I don't eat into small serving measured dishes and afterward microwave some for supper every night. In the event that your pot turns out to be colossal, you can make a twofold cluster.

Thai Green Curry Cook with a cup of Jasamine Rice (I actually have a 20lb sack I got for 13 bucks, American Long Grain sucks) Should be sufficient for 3 suppers with a 13.5oz can.

The pail of curry glue keeps going quite a while and costs 2 bucks, get coconut cream, get Chaokoh (This is by all accounts the best normal brand of coconut milk imho, and regularly have a solitary serving measured can, just would have to recalculate with that volume) on the off chance that you don't have a 99 Ranch close to you, (Their in store brand coconut cream is great and 60-70 pennies a can)

The fish sauce ensure you get one with a decent top regardless of anything else, a ton of the plastic ones simply keep opening up and you don't need your space to smell awful, yet fish sauce is utilized in a great deal of thai dishes. Likewise cook with thigh meat in case you're poor. I realize I regularly get bonless for 1.50-1.79 when it's discounted here a pound

In any case, it might cost a couple of bucks to get everything (around 6-7) however will be less expensive later on the grounds that you got the glue and fish sauce. It's truly scrumptious particularly with a rich coconut milk. The red curry on allrecipes isn't as acceptable, so in the event that I need a milder curry, I simply change out green curry glue for red curry glue. However, it's similarly tantamount to cafés and VASTLY not the same as what you'd get in the cafeteria.

Broccoli side dish:

- Chop some broccoli into sensible sizes, placed it into a giant bowl.

- Drizzle a tad of olive oil over it and throw to cover.

- Add a touch of salt, a ton of pepper, and a tad of sugar, throw again to cover. * Original formula calls for ~10 mins cooking in a stove at ~400F, yet I generally make a bit 'plate' out of aluminum foil and throw it on the BBQ for ~10 mins. Great and bravo, back off of the salt and sugar.

- Onions are modest and keep going quite a while. Green chime peppers will add to the flavor however aren't absolutely essential. They are tedious simply because it takes in any event an hour to cook down onions to cover something with.

Hack two onions (and one chime pepper in the event that you have it), clench hand size or bigger, as finely as could reasonably be expected. Take a 10" - 12" skillet with 3 Tbs of oil (veg, canola, olive) on medium warmth. Toss your onions (and chime pepper) in and let them cook. Mix them at regular intervals to ignite sure they don't. It takes about an hour to cook down two onions, don't be enticed to turn up the warmth however. Whenever they are cooked down altogether, include your meat. It very well may be swiss steak (too modest) or chicken or even hilshire ranch wiener, any meat will do. Cook the meat in the onions for 30 minutes, season with garlic powder and salt to taste. Serve over rice.

Salsa Chicken-

This is one of the most straightforward, least expensive, most beneficial methods of cooking chicken: prepare it in salsa. Put a chicken bosom in a pyrex dish, add a drop of olive oil, and afterward cover that thing in salsa. Allow it to heat at 350 until it smells pleasant and the focal point of the chicken isn't pink any longer. Tasty.

You can throw a yam in there on the rack over the chicken rack, and it'll cook and dribble onto the preparing sheet beneath it, and be truly delicious.

Miso Bowl-

My unsurpassed top pick, however this requires a stove:

Make some miso stock (protip - huge container of miso glue is modest, makes extraordinary amounts of heavenly soup). Line a bowl with aluminum foil, place a large portion of a block of ramen noodles in the middle. Add a few bits of fish, shrimp, other fish, whatever, alongside certain mushrooms, some bean stew pieces... fundamentally, anything you think would go great with the remainder of your fixings. Pour in the miso stock, add a touch of rice wine vinegar, wrap up the bundle, remove from the bowl, and spot in the broiler for a piece. You'll wind up steaming the entirety of your fixings so they cook actually pleasantly. Set the bundle back in your bowl, open up, eat.

It seems as though a ton, yet it truly isn't. I keep a cosco pack of frozen tilapia in my cooler, and it's an extraordinary method to make food a touch all the more fascinating. The other preferred position is that it doesn't need any washing. Wash the stock pot, clear off chopsticks, toss out foil.

FRITO PIE

Fixings: 1 jar of diced tomatoes 1 container of "stew starter" stew beans or stew beans and stew blend/sauce/whatever 1 lb of ground meat sack o fritos pack o sharp cheddar

- Brown and channel hamburger - Place meat beens and tomatoes into pot. Cover/stew for 7-10 minutes. - Put stew in a bowl with fritos and destroyed cheddar. blend it up a piece iwth your spoon and afterward appreciate. great with a glass of milk.

Noodles with nut sauce. Pasta is hella modest and you can add any meat you like. I substitute whichever meat is marked down at Vons in the half off rack.

Nut Sauce:

1 cup of nutty spread. 1-2 tablespon of rice vinegar, however other vinegar works, 1 tablespoon of seasame oil, however different oils work, 2 tablespoons of soy sauce, 1-2 tablespoon sugar. Change things dependent on your inclinations.

Simply combine these all and pour onto the noodles after they've been stressed. I like to add shrimp so I simply throw them in with the bubbling noodles for 5 minutes and they are cooked.

Lightning Source UK Ltd.
Milton Keynes UK
UKHW021030080121
376609UK00001B/2